Get Fit, Healthy and Staying That Way, 40+

A Beginner's Guide to Fitness and Why it Doesn't Require a Midlife Crisis

By

Norman Brown, Personal Trainer

My goals:

Write your own goals below. Make them specific, measurable, attainable, relevant and in time blocks

Keep a copy on your fridge, another on your mobile phone and anywhere else you always look.

My Personal Message to You

Here's my personal message to you, from the author - Norman Brown. That's me here!

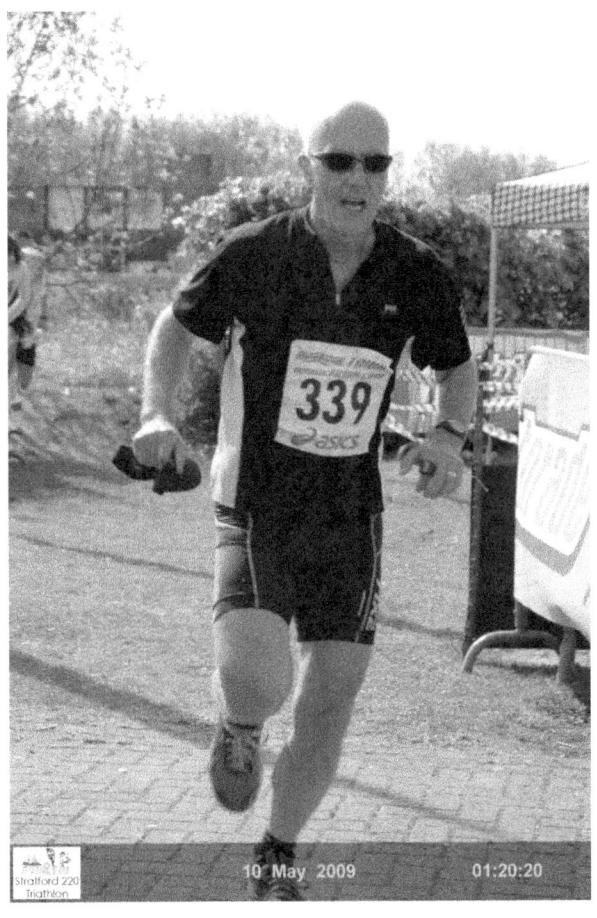

Are you being hassled to start to exercise, confused by all the conflicting information on diet and exercise and how it affects your life expectancy?

I fully understand where you're coming from. I've been there, got the t-shirt and learned from being unable to walk one hundred yards without being out of breath - to running marathons, triathlons and competing in mountain running challenges.

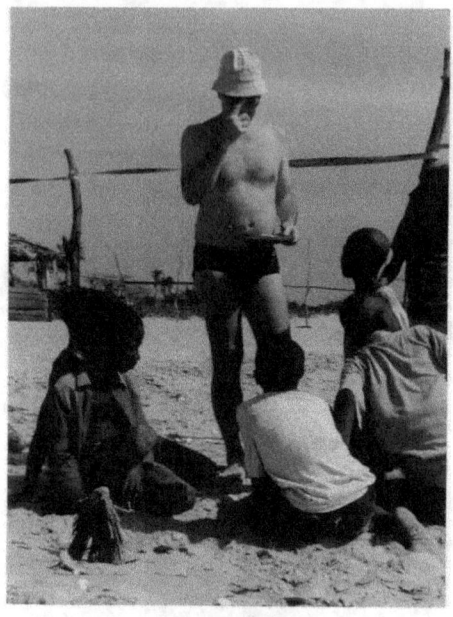

My overweight days...

This book will explain, in simple terms, just how easy it is to approach exercise in midlife. It is not as daunting or complicated as it appears. This book is a beginner's guide to exercise if you are over 40 and not (currently) exercising (enough).

If there's anything you don't understand as you're reading through, for example, the names and explanations of different exercises, you'll find a number of easy descriptions as you read through the book.

You do NOT need to reach my high level of fitness, as a personal trainer, at age 65+. It is a great target to meet and beat.

You **CAN**, however, reach the level of fitness that suits **you**, **your** health and future wellbeing.

"Physical fitness is not only one of the most important keys to a healthy body, it is the basis of dynamic and creative intellectual activity."

John F. Kennedy

Contents

Dedication

"This book is dedicated to the memory of **Ken McGregor** - a fine friend and inspiration to all who knew him."

About The Author - Norman Brown

Why Me - And - Why Should You Consider Anything I Have To Say About Fitness And Training?

I came into the fitness industry late in my life, at 52, after a long career in hospitality as a development manager. A career in hospitality invariably involved lots of entertaining, long hours and more often than not, plenty of stress.

My career span during the early 70's and 80's was a time when smoking and excess alcohol was quite normal and the only exercise was walking the kids to school.

Gradually, my weight increased and by the time I reached my late 40's stress levels became so high I thought I was having a heart attack.

In fact, I rocked up at A&E one day thinking the worse was to be told to me. I was only having a stress attack and was told to go and lose some weight! No nonsense back then.

This kicked my butt and I started to think about my lifestyle and it was time to go for a run. Huh! The first run I made was a 0.9 mile lap and I had to stop 6 times to gather my breath, I was so unfit.

I was determined to make a change so I stuck at it three times a week. The only training advice I had received was from reading the magazine 'Runners World,' and you know, it worked.

Just 2 years later, I ran my first marathon in 4.06.57. I ran 10 miles in 60 minutes 1 year later and so far I have run over 300 races from 10k to 55 mile ultras.

I was so hooked on my successes that I changed my career to that of a personal trainer and now spend all my time helping people like you to improve your fitness and change your lifestyle and overall wellbeing.

It is the most valuable and priceless change I made in my life since getting married and my wife agrees!

I have seen an enormous development in the fitness industry in the past few years, but unfortunately, I have also witnessed the enormous growth of obesity in men and women of all ages.

In the last 12 years I have assessed, coached and personal trained hundreds of people through all manner of lifestyle and medical conditions.

This does not make me a medical expert, but it has prepared me to advise you on the most common of lifestyle conditions which will help you make significant improvements to your routines, health and fitness.

I have been fortunate enough to have worked and be trained by one of the UK's best independent health providers. They possess an unrivalled track record in clinically governed recommendations.

My personal record of achievements includes:

> 35 Full marathons with a personal best (PB) of 3:18
> 4 Ultra marathons in Switzerland and the UK
> Over 200 short distance races including half marathons PB 1:27
> Olympic Triathlons age group winner when I was 60
> 3 British 4 peaks; race finisher in the top 6
> 6 Half iron man distance completed in some of the UK's hardest terrains.

There is so much education available to everyone (you're holding most of what you need in your hands just now), yet we do not appear to get the general message across to enough people to make a big enough difference throughout our communities and society in general.

I have seen many who have decided to increase their fitness and training for the benefit of their long term health – and you can join them and benefit in the days, weeks, months and years ahead – with successful, habit forming ideas. I have helped to effectively change their fitness and behaviours, to alter their lifestyles – for the better.

I am extremely hopeful that this book will help you to achieve the changes you want for yourself. Good luck.

Important Legal Disclaimer

Before you do anything, begin any new physical training, exercise, please read and act upon the following:

The subsequent information reflects the author's opinions and does **NOT** replace advice from a medical professional.

BEFORE beginning this or any exercise program, please first consult a physician to ensure that it's appropriate for you. The author has attempted to provide accurate information in this publication, but accepts no responsibility for any damages or losses of any kind that may occur as a result of actions taken after reviewing the contents of this work. The reader assumes 100% responsibility for the use of part, any and all information contained within the text.

How to Use This Book

Using This Book

If you are new to exercising and not sure how to approach it then I would recommend spending some time reading the first few pages to understand where to start safely. If you have some idea and looking to compare my advice with your own experience you can just jump straight to the relevant chapter which is relevant to you.

I have deliberately left the exercising programme ideas towards the end because the main purpose of this book is to provide you with a framework with which to start preparing you for a transformation programme which can be measured; progressed - then success!

Introduction

Congratulations, if you are looking at this book with a view to starting to exercise. This is already a major step forward and you should feel proud of this achievement. Often, we, as busy individuals, go through the first stages of our lives building careers and homes at the expense of our personal wellbeing.

This is quite normal until one day, when something happens to make you realise you have been too busy to look after yourself. This may be a photograph showing you have spread a little. It could be stress from work or a serious health incident that takes you to your local A&E. Any of these could be pushing your button. Whatever it is, it's never too late!

I plan to explain how easy it is for you to improve your current health status, simplify exercise and eat healthier, mostly a little at a time and at a speed that suits you best.

By following a few set guidelines I can help you work out where you are right now. This begins with arranging a health check with your GP to check you are fit enough to take the first steps.

I expect you will have heard it all before and maybe your health is okay, but are you sure? There are medical signs which will determine how you will exercise at the correct intensity and with the best choice of exercise for you.

I don't say this lightly, as after 14 years of carrying out pre-exercise assessments I have helped to identify high blood pressure, high glucose, high cholesterol levels, low body weight and high body weight.

In one case I remember an individual came to see me early one morning with a pale complexion and not feeling well. After checking his blood pressure we recommended he went straight to A&E where he ended up having a triple bypass. I didn't complete the bypass for him, but without it...

We know there is a health crisis across the world, primarily in western heavily commercialised countries.

After the spread of developing social, economic and financial wealth, this has caused us to develop transport infrastructure to move us and food around the world. Food manufacturing must cater for the overwhelming clamber for fast (and easy to prepare) food.

This has resulted in people moving less and consuming more sugar than could ever be dreamed of in the 1950's and 60's when those same populations were less fat, had far fewer diabetes difficulties and considerable less heart disease.

Testimonial

"Hi Norman,

I have always been big as are the majority of my family. Most of my family have diabetes and two years ago we received the news that my brother had died, (age 53) from not looking after his diabetes. My father also died young (age 49) and I didn't want to end up the same. I wanted to be around to see my nieces and nephews grow up and have their own families.

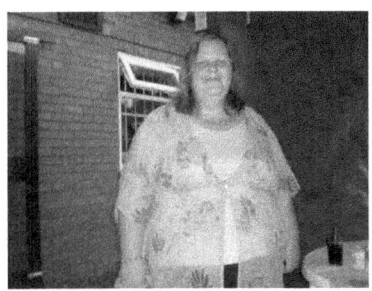

The before "picture"

I knew I had to do something. In October 2013 I did "Stoptober" and gave up cigarettes. I then used some of the money that I would of spent on cigarettes to join Nuffield Fitness Centre in February.

To be honest, I have not looked back since; with the help of all the staff there and the support of my husband, friends and family. I have managed to loose 4st so far.

I am still learning new ways of exercising and enjoy it, having a mentor and joining the "slim to win" group and joining in with classes has helped me to learn more about different types of exercise.

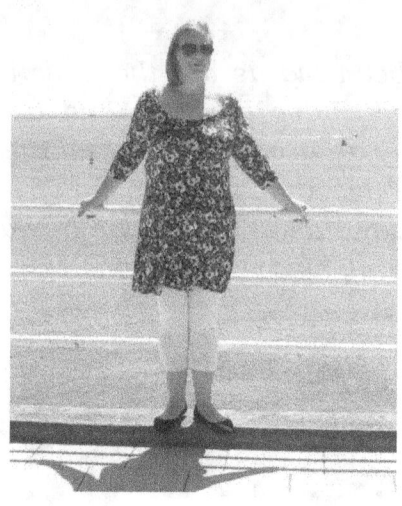

The after "picture"

My health has improved now and I have more confidence in myself. I am finding that I can do things that I wouldn't have been able to do before.

Susan"

The Health Risks & Why You Need to Change

The next short passage may be a little technical, but is important to understand so you can plan ahead properly.

Cardiovascular Disease (CVD)

In the U.S. Cardiovascular disease affects 65 million Americans. Close to one million Americans have a heart attack each year?

In the U.S. one person dies of cardiovascular disease every 39 seconds; that's 1 million deaths of Americans each year.

Cardiovascular Disease in the UK

In 2011 there were 160,000 deaths; 74,000 were a direct cause of coronary heart disease - the UK's biggest killer. Source [NHS-UK][WHO][Kesser]

Prevention Top Tips

1. Where you are overweight; lose weight.
2. Should you have a poor diet; improve it.

The risk of CVD is increased greatly when you are overweight, of poor fitness and not exercising regularly, increasing the risk of white blood cells hooking up with bad cholesterol and blocking the arteries over time. This may cause a heart attack or a stroke.

When we were kids, we were given fish oils, in the form of castor oil. This is still one of the most effective ways to reduce fatty plaque build-up in your arteries.

The (re)introduction to your diet of oily fish and other omega 3 sources like nuts, dairy and red meats is a good way to increase your omega 3's and reduce your risk of a heart attack.

Metabolic Syndrome

Metabolic syndrome is becoming increasingly common. It occurs when a range of metabolic risk factors such as obesity and insulin resistance come together.

Metabolic syndrome increases your risk of developing type 2 diabetes.

A number of alternative terms exist to describe the condition, such as syndrome X, Reaven's syndrome and in Australia, CHAOS.

1 in 3 Americans have metabolic syndrome; a cluster of major cardiovascular risk factors related to being overweight/obese and with insulin resistance.

The total cost of cardiovascular disease in 2008 was estimated at $300 billion. Source: [Kesser]

Diabetes

The World Health Organisation (WHO) projects that diabetes will be the 7th leading cause of death by 2030.

In 2012, 29.1 million Americans, or 9.3% of the population, had diabetes. 2010, the figures were 25.8 million and 8.3%.
Of the 29.1 million, 21.0 million were diagnosed, and 8.1 million were undiagnosed. In 2010 the figures were 18.8 million and 7.0 million

In 2010 there were 1.7 million new diagnoses per year; in 2012 this increased to 1.9 million.
Source: [diabetes.org]

In the UK

There are about 3.7 million people with diabetes including an estimated 850,000 people who are undiagnosed.
Source [diabetes UK]

Diagnosing Diabetes

The symptoms of diabetes are passing urine more often than usual - especially at night; increased thirst; extreme tiredness; unexplained weight loss; genital itching or regular episodes of thrush; slow healing of cuts and wounds; and - blurred vision.

Type 1 Diabetes develops when the insulin-producing cells in the body have been destroyed and the body is unable to produce any insulin at all.

Everyone with Type 1 diabetes has to be treated with insulin. The symptoms are usually very obvious and develop very quickly, especially in children. It's important to emphasise here that type 1 diabetes is often confused by people who don't understand the condition. Type 1 diabetes occurs and generally affects individuals early in life.

For Type 2 diabetes, signs are less obvious and often develop over some years. Type 2 diabetes is a lifestyle condition. This is why it is often diagnosed following a routine medical check later in life.

The Biggest Diabetes Risk Factors Are:

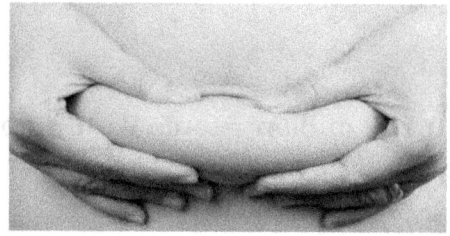

1. You are overweight with a large waist or
2. You have a close relative with the condition; or
3. You are from a black or South Asian background

The World Health Organisation (WHO) recommends:
a healthy diet; regular physical activity; maintaining a normal body weight and avoiding tobacco use - and suggests that these can prevent or delay the onset of type 2 diabetes (4)

That's enough about All the Scary Stuff.

I would like to concentrate on the physical and what you can do to offset the scary parts – and share with you how to make some serious changes for your long term better health and exercising support for the rest of your life.

"The typical response from people when I tell them I'm diabetic is, 'Oh, I'm sorry to hear that.' You know, I'm not. I'm a better athlete because of diabetes rather than despite it. I'm more aware of my training, my fitness and more aware of nutrition. I'm more proactive about my health."

Charlie Kimball

A Cautionary Note on Posture

If you are new to exercise it will be beneficial to take professional advice from a registered qualified trainer, to instruct you in using and maintaining the correct posture when using (heavy or heavier) weights.

It's pretty well impossible to be sure that you are capable of using good posture if you have not been instructed previously. Almost every client I see needs corrective training to improve how they move safely.

Good body position is fundamental to improving how you move every day. Getting instruction will ensure you exercise safely, improve muscle activation, get better at lifting and pushing your body around and also lifting weights more efficiently. This will help you with picking up your shopping, moving your bed, your washing machine and any heavy gardening activities.

Getting Started: Steps to Success

What Is Your Current Health Like?

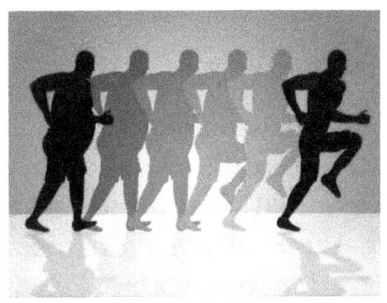

Before you begin an exercise programme you should consider your current health status. Where you have been inactive and may be overweight; have any health conditions or a history of heart related conditions in your family, always seek the advice of your doctor.

Your health status will fall into a number of categories:

➢ Normal Green; which means you have no significant health issues that need to be taken into consideration.
➢ Caution 1 Amber; you may have slightly higher BMI / BP / glucose or cholesterol levels requiring you to take a moderate approach.
➢ Caution 2 Amber; you may have high BP/ chest pains / physical conditions which challenge what you can do, so you may have to take a much more careful approach to your plan including using a physiotherapist and/or

a personal trainer, to ensure you exercise cautiously and within strict guidelines.

"Please understand that the majority of health related conditions are improved by exercise."

Why Is Exercise So Important In The First Place?

The body is designed to move and to move you need oxygen. The less efficient your cardiovascular system is, the more difficult it will be to move around; let alone play with the kids, run in the park, or cycle. If your muscles are weak you may be or become unstable, which can mean you are more likely to fall and damage your skeletal system.

If you have been inactive for a long time your blood cholesterol may be higher than normal which can lead to atherosclerosis, which if ignored and untreated, can cause artery blockages leading to angina, heart attack or stroke.

"High blood pressure can be improved by gradually exercising more and adhering to a healthy diet."

Depression

Recent research has highlighted that people who are physically active in their leisure time were less likely to suffer from depression, with every weekly session of activity reducing the overall risks. A University College London study found that those who exercised three times weekly could lower their risk of becoming depressed by 16 per cent.

I hope you can now see that exercise is at the very route of improving almost all conditions which are currently holding you back and putting your health now and in the future, at an increased risk of a wide range of extreme problems.

"The purpose of training is to tighten up the slack, toughen the body, and polish the spirit."

Morihei Ueshiba

Warning: A Toxic Relationship with Exercise

This is long, but it's very important to read this through.

A personal account by Carol

"I'm glad to say that now, exercise and I are good friends and have a healthy relationship with no needy dependencies, but it wasn't always like that!

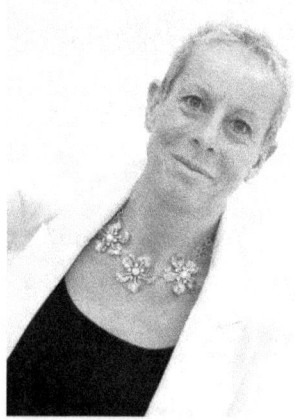

As a kid at senior school I detested anything that remotely resembled physical exercise. Being overweight and having excruciatingly poor hand to eye co-ordination did nothing to help encourage a love of sport which was largely based on team ball sports.

My passion for exercise emerged when, recently married, I decided to take up running. Sadly, this also coincided with my very unhealthy attitude towards my now svelte size and being diagnosed borderline anorexic. Running, I claimed, was for fitness and de-stressing, but what I wasn't admitting was that it was a coping mechanism enabling me to maintain some level of normal eating as I saw it as the way to simply burn off the calories. For twenty years, barely a day passed when I didn't get out pounding the streets – hurricanes (yes I ran the morning after the great storm in 1987), snow, ice, heat; none of it mattered. My trainers came on every holiday we took and if I missed a day's run I was tense and miserable. I broke my wrist one winter, while ice-skating – that didn't stop me running – it was my wrist for heaven's sake not my leg or ankle! One year I ended up in A&E two days before Christmas when I'd cut my hand very badly – later that day I was out pounding the icy lanes on an 8 mile run.

I also got into aerobics as the craze swept the country in the early 1980s – star jumps, grapevines etc., became my world for at least two hours a week. When aerobics gave way to step I was one of the early devotees eager to use high blocks, hand weights and ankle weights to improve my cardio fitness and stamina. During the 1990s when I first ran my own business it also revolved around my exercise routines. A run in the morning, followed by a swim, were standard practice Monday-Saturday and a step class every evening with two classes on a Saturday were just part of the daily routine. It never occurred to me that I was doing any damage (to my mind and body) and when people advised me to take rest days I'd nod indulgently and not have any intention to follow their advice.

My world hit a reality wall in 1997 when I fell off my step during a class, tearing tendons and ligaments in my ankle.

I'd never known so much pain and it took three months before I was pain free, and probably would have been less if I'd not been so impatient to get back to exercise!

Finally in 2003 I had to give up running – I'd been getting pains in my hips and my ITB (Iliotibial band. An ITB friction syndrome is a common injury to the knee) were tight for months and no amount of stretching seemed to ease them out. I was literally pulled up short on a run when I couldn't physically move my legs any more. I had to admit that there was a problem and the start of years of treatment, while physiotherapists and specialists tried to get to the bottom of what was wrong. On top of conventional physiotherapy I tried controversial blood injections in my hamstrings, cortisone injections into my spine under MRI, I wore a pelvic belt, travelled to Harley Street and saw a number of different specialists. During all of this time I had to adapt my exercise routine and swimming became my nemesis. I dropped classes for over three years and when I did return swapped the high intensity aerobics for body conditioning. I trained much more in the gym, but was prone to long bouts on cardio machines, though I did try to vary my routines.

The body conditioning classes were great with an excellent instructor who focused very hard on core strength and the correct posture, but for me it was starting to work with a personal trainer that was the real turning point for me. I'd known Richard (Cowell) for years as I'd attended his step and aerobic classes, so when we talked over a coffee and I explained all of the treatment I'd been having and how I wanted to get fitter and stronger he agreed to help, first talking to my physiotherapist and getting a good understanding of what I'd been through. Now 6 years later Richard's still training me, we meet in the gym twice a week and I balance this with body conditioning, combat and

Zumba classes, and walking with my dogs. I'm not entirely free of aches and pain. My pelvis is weak on the left and sometimes gets out of position, needing physiotherapy to rectify (the problem). My left hamstring still has a tendency to tighten up when I've overdone it and I have to be careful to ensure I don't sit (still) for long periods of time as I stiffen up anywhere between my lower back and hamstrings. Long car journeys can be agony whether I'm a passenger or driver, even with an automatic (transmission), but when I'm having a good period I can manage these with ease. I take these aches and pains very much as the price I've paid for not listening to my body for years and accept them as minor ailments and live with them.

As for diet – it took about 20 years before I could say that I was free of the anorexia, but now I have a much healthier relationship with food and do not panic if I put on the odd pound, knowing that it's normal to fluctuate a bit and that it doesn't actually matter. If I miss a class then it's a shame, but not something that I'm going to go to pieces over and insist that I miss a meal to compensate.

I have never been fitter or had better core strength. My body shape has changed and I often get comments about my upper body muscle definition. I'm a toned size 8-10, aged 52, who loves exercise for the benefits it gives me and not as a means to being able to eat!

Carol

Carol is an ex customer of mine from my previous working life, at the restaurant - Shaker Brown.

Exercise: What It Means For You

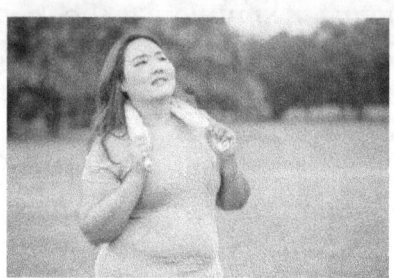

Fitness is a relative term used to describe what you want or what to expect from yourself in terms of being physically fit. This is often judged by you, when comparing yourself with someone else who you consider to be fitter than you. Hey, this could put unrealistic pressure on you, so think about what it means to be fit - for you. The first thing to consider is what improved fitness will look like for you.

Age Related Exercise

Fitness, whether you're 50 or 90, is a good thing. There is little to worry about if you follow these sensible guidelines. Exercising moderately will improve your lifestyle, by reducing many health risks such as Type 2 diabetes, cancers, obesity, osteoporosis, high blood pressure and also reduce your risk of heart attack and strokes.

Other good fitness benefits include reducing artery atherosclerosis by increasing your good cholesterol, through diet and exercise. As your fitness improves you will strengthen your heart, helping to deliver more oxygen to your muscles. In turn this will help you to perform everyday activities with considerably more energy.

Reducing your stress levels, through exercising, will improve your ability to deal with difficult decisions more easily at work or at home - and increase your productivity.

You will sleep better and be more relaxed due to increases in hormone activity, such as serotonin, which aides sleep. Achieving a good night's sleep will balance your energy and control hunger hormones and see you waking more refreshed, every morning.

Look around you and you may notice that people who do not exercise are often over weight and suffering the effects of long term lifestyle diseases and conditions associated with little or no activity. Those you see who are older and moving around more easily are generally of normal weight and have always exercised or at least been active during their lives.

I regularly see people at the gym, in their 70's and 80's, enjoying their exercise as well as anyone half their age. The oldest member of my gym was 91 when he passed away sadly this year of natural causes, but he came to the gym 3 times a week - which helped prolong and improve his quality of life.

60 is now considered the new 40 as people are now living longer and many over 100 years of age. The reality of a better quality of life needs to be recognised and grasped if you are to enjoy your retirement.

Activity Choices

Before we go to deep into exercise and what that will mean for you, many people just don't like the idea of the conventional concept of exercise. There are other options. Not all sports have to be as rough and tumble as rugby or as all-consuming as marathon running. There are plenty of gentler activities that you can take up at any age, which will allow you to reap health benefits alongside the pleasure that comes from mastering a new skill and making new friends.

Golf

Playing requires strength, power, flexibility, balance, core stability, body awareness, and endurance. They're all physical traits that every golfer must possess.

Tai Chi

Practicing the ancient art of Tai Chi can improve your fitness through this slow-moving exercise which is hugely popular in the Far East and is increasingly practiced by people around the world in a bid to improve balance, strength and flexibility.

Yoga

This ancient form of exercise focuses on strength, flexibility and breathing to boost physical and mental wellbeing. The main components of yoga are postures (a series of movements designed to increase strength and flexibility) and breathing.

Paddle Boarding

If you live near the coast or a lake, paddle boarding can offer you lots of benefits to improve your cardio vascular fitness and deliver strength, flexibility, balance and coordination.

Table Tennis

Fun and also great cardiovascular exercise, with little injury risk, or strain on the joints and you can choose the intensity at which you want to play.

Fencing

Developed into a sport in the 18th century and now practiced worldwide. It can be found in regional centres. In most areas this involves training skills which require great coordination, balance and core strength.

Dancing

Dance is the UK's fastest growing art form. More than 4.8 million people regularly attend community dance groups each year, in England, alone.

Whether you like to jump or jive, tap or tango, shake your belly or your booty, dancing is one of the most enjoyable ways to get some exercise.

Swimming

As a really great exercise to work the whole body in a comfortable environment, you have the additional benefits of buoyancy to support you from any impact issues if you are rehabilitating from injury. Your weight prevents you from any impact exercise, so you can improve your cardio vascular system as well as work on flexibility. Your class choices include aqua classes in swimming pools which are extremely popular with anyone who does not wish to flash the flesh in a gym.

The point I want to make is that not all exercise has to be boring or based in the gym. There are so many ways to engage in a new activity and all have the following benefits: stronger heart, improved flexibility, stronger core, better coordination and strength, all of which are shown to reduce your risk of most of the common life threatening conditions.

"The reason I exercise is for the quality of life I enjoy."

Kenneth H. Cooper

Determine What Your Goal Is

There are more potential goals than I can list here, so try these for a start:

1. I want to lose weight. Okay, how much?
2. I want to improve fitness. What does that mean? Walk 30 minutes without stopping or run a 5K race in under 30 minutes?
3. I want to improve my cholesterol level. From what to what?
4. Control my blood sugar. What figures do you want?
5. Get stronger. How will you measure the change?
6. Improve my weight. From what to what?
7. Put muscle weight on. How much and where?

These are all popular choices and you now need to drill down and decide what, why, in what time and decide if it is realistic.

The best targets are small ones which you can achieve in a month, with each as minor steps towards larger, long term targets.

Once you decide on your targets, write them inside, on page 2 of this book, as a reminder and a prompt to 'stick to it.'

How to Assess Your Progress

This will be completed in a number of ways, so let's go through how to chart and manage your progress.

First, decide the best way to measure any improvement. This will depend on your goal. I will offer a couple of examples which you can adapt to your personal targets:

Walking

Keep a diary of how far you walk and record the times (length of the walk). This works wonderfully for your motivation as you see yourself getting out more often and for longer.

Weight Loss

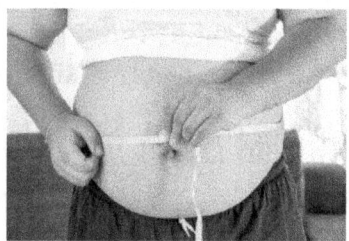

This is my personal favourite. Most people confuse weight loss targets with their total weight. Stop immediately - it's different. The body is made up of skeletal bones, lean muscle, fat and water.

You can't accurately assume that what you lose each week is either fat or water, or the total, because they all interact.

As you lose body fat, your body may increase lean muscle and water, so you think you're not losing weight, but you are. Time will prove this to you.

The easiest method to check this is to use real and accurate tape measurements of key positions around your body;

1. Chest, under or over the breast, or midline of nipples for gents
2. Abdominal, on the line of your navel
3. Hips, at the largest point
4. Upper thigh, at the largest point
5. Mid-calf
6. Upper arm
7. Lower arm

Total up the inches or centimetres and keep a record each time you repeat the measurement, say monthly or every Saturday morning. This will give you a true reflection of your body fat loss, which is the most important one to improve.

If your goal is to put weight on because you are under weight, then I recommend much the same as fat loss. Record your measurements and also your weight changes. Except this time you are looking to make sure you are gaining lean and not body fat.

Using and monitoring with a set of body fat scales is the best way of checking your weight gain. If you don't have scales you can use a tape measure and look for a change in the dimensions around your limbs, particularly around your waste-line. At the same time, watch your body fat does not increase too greatly. You are looking for muscle growth over weeks and months, not days.

For improving fitness: if you are unfit, but capable of a jog, I recommend finding yourself a route of around 3k to 5k and time your run once a week. Each week, see if it improves. Use your diary to record all your daily runs to ensure you are getting out. Once a week, record the time, distance and your heart rate.

Checking your heart rate (how hard your heart is working, pumping blood around your body) is the most accurate way to assess your effort levels for the improving exerciser, which is important if you have high blood pressure. You should exercise at around 70% of your heart rate (HR) maximum.

Calculating your exercising heart rate is pretty easy (220 – Your Age) x 70, will give you your approximate maximum HR. Multiply this number by 70% for moderate exercising. (If you require a more accurate measure and are in good health you should consult a trainer or coach to perform a Maximum heart rate test, for most new exercisers though this formula for calculating 70% is usually sufficient) Measuring your heart rate is the most accurate way to assess if you are training at an appropriate effort level for your current level of fitness. Training too hard with a high heart rate may suggest that you may be over training. This applies particularly in the case of someone with (known or unknown) cardio vascular problems or is suffering with high blood pressure.

Important:

In these situations you should be maintaining lower effort levels meaning you should still be able to talk easily.

If you are training to improve your fitness with no health concerns, using a heart rate monitor will ensure you keep within your goal training heart rate (HR) minimum and maximum zones.

Heart rate monitors can become an essential piece of equipment to keep you on track, much the same way as a tachometer or speedometer in your car. Would you go out for a drive without reading your speedo? Exercise should be no different.

You can get HR monitors on your phone, wrist bands and chest bands, working with a wide range of wrist monitors. If you are just starting out you do not need anything too clever. Keep it simple and go for a basic model and if you are a regular exerciser, choose one which suits your sport, because they are all amazingly specific.

What Else Can You Do?

If you really want to make an impact on your life, you will need to think about understanding how weight training can impact on all your improvements.

The very mention of weight training to most people new to exercise is scary to say the least. It is confusing. Beefing up and competition are things I am not interested in and are not what I am talking about!

Not at all; period.

Well, this is time to wake up and smell the coffee. Weight training for you is definitely nothing like the stereo type images you might have in your mind right now.

What is Resistance Exercise?

Simply, this is moving your body against resistance. This can be one or all of the following basic movements and preferably a combination of them all.

Pushing; Pulling; Squatting; Lifting; Pressing.

This is not difficult. Anyone can do this and you probably carry out some forms of resistance already every day, in some ways. To make this pattern into a routine depends on how fit you are at the start. This is why you need to test and record your current strength.

Weight training can be accomplished in so many ways. If you are new with this training, start with your own body weight by gently squatting and completing push-ups.

Here's how all are completed for either 30 seconds, or 1 minute, if you are quite unfit.

1. Squat down as far as you can, standing push your hips back and continue to squat down by hinging from your knee, heels stay on the floor with your thighs parallel to the floor, your knees should be behind or in line with your feet, and make a note of the angle if you can't get all the way down. Record how many you can do in a minute. Alternatively sit in a chair and stand up and sit down X times in the minute.

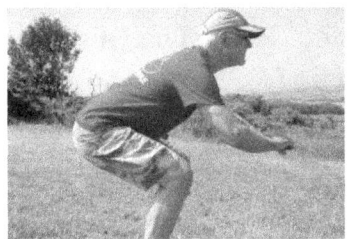

2. Press-ups, lay on the floor and place your hands just outside your shoulders, push your heels back and attempt to lift your whole body off the floor, as many times as you can in the time.

   Struggling, then bring up your knees and cantilever from the knee until your chest touches the floor.

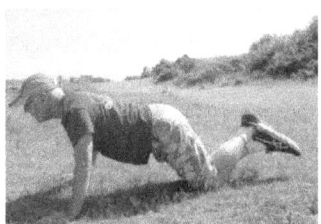

3. Shoulder Press, using hand weights or anything as simple as a sports bag full of sand, lifting it off the floor and repeatedly pressing above your head until your arms feel like lead and you can't do another one! Record the result and the weight you used.

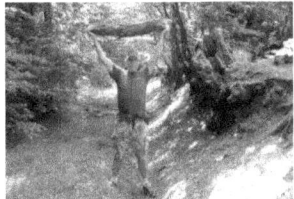

Record these in the front of your training diary and recheck and compare monthly.

Exercise, Involving Resistance, Has The Following Benefits:

Accelerates fat loss; by increasing your metabolism following any strength exercises. Basically, as you exercise with weights you are breaking down muscle tissue. Upon completion of your weight exercises your body needs to repair by rebuilding tissue.

During this phase your energy system will be metabolizing fat for fuel. As this phase can last for several hours more than cardio vascular training, it is a far more efficient method for losing fat weight.

Builds lean muscle; we all need to protect our lean muscle, particularly as we age, when we tend to lose muscle. Weight training, therefore, will help to protect your lean mass for the following reason; as you rebuild tissue you are improving strength and replacing weakened tissue with stronger muscle fibres.

The effects of ageing on muscles facts that you should be aware of:

Loss of muscle strength is a process that starts around age 30 and can be as high as 30% at 50 and progresses throughout life. By 70, your muscle loss can be 50%. In this process, the amount of muscle tissue and the number and size of muscle fibres gradually decrease.

The result is a gradual loss of muscle mass and muscle strength. This mild loss of muscle strength places increased stress on certain joints (such as the knees) and may predispose a person to arthritis or falling.

Fortunately, the loss in muscle mass and strength can partially be overcome or at least significantly delayed by a program of regular exercise including resistance training. Muscles are not able to contract as quickly in old age.

As you improve strength you are also activating a greater percentage of muscle fibres which enable you to improve balance and perform every day activities with greater safety. Improved posture will reduce the stress on your body. You will also feel less tired.

"A muscle is like a car. If you want it to run well early in the morning, you have to warm it up."

Florence Griffith Joyner

Tracking Your Exercise and Lifestyle Changes

By tracking your exercise and lifestyle particularly, all the detail is important to help keep yourself motivated at times when you are not sure if your efforts are working. Where you are putting in the time, your effort will pay off.

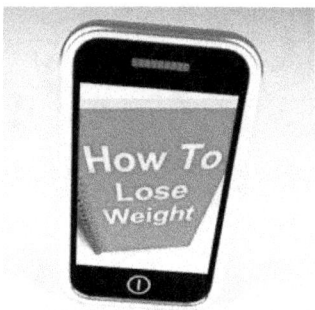

There are many ways you can track everything in your life now. In the exercise and health world they are called "wearables." You can get an app to track exercise, activity, health and nutrition.

They are a great way for you to keep on top of the changes you have decided are necessary for putting you in control of your own life changing recreation.

There are many choices, from a simple phone app for heart rate monitors recording time, heart rate, energy output (calories,) to those which will break down your exercise activity to pace and time per mile and elevation. Where you are using GPS, you can set intervals on a particular course you use, so you can compare previous efforts by yourself or others.

I highly recommend you consider tracking your exercise. Choose an app appropriate for your type of activity; running, swimming, cycling etc. All have their own unique tracking measurements.

As a general exerciser, you only need something simple. There is a wide choice.

The simplest way to track your effort levels is with a paper diary which you can look back on in a few months and marvel at the changes and accomplishments you have made as a result of all of your hard work.

Why?

Whatever your occupation or profession, if you are to succeed you need to set yourself goals/targets. These goals are broken down into smaller achievable tasks. This will help keep you on track.

Sticking to the plan is important.

Your choice of tracking device can help you by making it easy to record your activities and see if and when you are going off your plan. I don't want you missing out on achieving the goal you are about to set.

The whole point here is to see that you are successful.

You can achieve success by:

1. Setting your goal/target
2. Organising your lifestyle to fit in your chosen changes
3. Breakdown your goal into monthly and weekly targets
4. Start tracking from day one

Motivation

Your motivation all depends on what made you read this training and exercise book in the first place. When your reason is strong enough you can start an exercise frequency appropriate to your current fitness level.

Here's other people's motivation:

- I have clients recovering from Cardiac surgery who won't miss a session
- A couple have a goal to get into shape for their wedding
- One lady is determined to lose 8 stone and on target; trains with me twice a week
- A gentleman who is underweight and needs to put on muscle to maintain good health and improve his strength.
- The lady who suffers from MS and trains once a week because she can't manage on her own
- Active exercisers who wish to improve their competitive edge

These are just a few individual motivations to give you an idea and dispel any myth, that as personal trainers, we only train healthy people or those with lots of money to burn. The facts are that training is as personal as having your hair done; it costs less and achieves great results for the right reasons.

Start now and improve your health and fitness for you and the family.

A Word or Two about Targeting Your Personal Best (PBs)

Should you always chase your personal best targets? You have to be realistic. For some, just staying active as many days a week as possible is a goal, which is why people tend to take up yoga, tai chi, walking and golf as they age.

You maintain the competitive edge by checking your results within age categories. This is where you set your age related goal. It's important to remain practical considering the age related recovery required. You can still aim high. You won't be quite as fast and you may need longer to recover. Importantly, you will give your best and not ever give up.

Even Usain Bolt won't be running the 100 metres in under ten seconds when he's 55 years old.

Enjoy every day you never know when the last will be.

Your Options for Exercise

Frequency

The official general guideline is currently 30 minutes of continuous exercise, 5 days a week.

I have a rule. It's simple; - **EXERCISE EVERY DAY.**

If you miss a day for an appointment it's not the end of the world, but if you only exercise for 3 days a week and drop a day for that appointment, you have lost over 33% of your week's training.

Believe me, you won't make it up.

Don't believe the excuse that you can't fit it in. You can.

You need to change your mind set to the one that says **"When am I going to exercise today?"**

Where to Exercise?

Here are a few suggestions, some obvious and others not so. Not all environments must be formal or expensive.

The Park

In your local park you will probably find a number of exercise groups. Ask for details and join in. Jogging, fitness classes, buggy groups, boot camps and walking; they are all there.

Swimming

In a pool, in the lake or in the sea are all available and mostly free. Some areas will have lifeguards to keep an eye on safety.

Community Halls

These almost always have a regular number of fitness classes where you can enrol.

Health Clubs/the Gym

This is where you will find structured facilities and coaches who will induct you into exercise. They will set you up with a basic program to begin with. As I stated previously, they vary in levels of service, so have a look to make sure you find something that works for you and ask friends and family that you trust, for recommendations with success stories.

One important consideration is how close the gym is to where you live or work? This will determine how likely you are to stay with them after your 'honeymoon' period has expired. If you have to drive past the facility each day you are more likely to make the effort, following a busy day.

Beware, that if you go home first you are much less likely to turn out again for the gym and miss a vital workout!

What About The Facilities You May Use?

The obvious one is open the door and enjoy the great outdoors, walking the block into your local park and discover just how much you can do either on your own, with a group, or with your partner.

The Gym; source a gym and select one which suits both your budget and your needs. This could be a subject on its own, but I will try to give you an idea of what to expect from your chosen facility (gym, leisure centre, etc.) From one which offers a high quality service and will cost more per month to a budget choice that generally has much less in the way of services, appearance and comfort.

There are a huge number of facilities looking for your business so take your time to visit and try out a guest day (often free or low cost.) This is the only way to assess if it's your kind of place to go to several times a week.

The gym is going to become a close friend; choose your friends carefully. The rule of thumb is the cheaper they are, the less service you will see and experience, which is fine when you are an experienced exerciser, but not so good if you need help and support.

You should assess the facilities for suitability to match the training you wish to do, at the times you can visit, by asking questions of the gym management and real (regular) users:

- How busy will it be when you will be training?

- Can you expect queues for the most popular equipment?
- What advice will you receive?
- Are there additional costs for this support?
- Will you receive an induction?
- Will you receive an assessment at the beginning and be provided with a program to follow with regular follow up if you need it?
- What is their personal training policy? My pet hate is personal trainers badgering for business and giving you a hard time when all you want to do is train. Personal training is a very effective service, but you should not feel obligated to buy their service. If you want to consider it, that's okay and I recommend a trainer, but go by reputation and recommendation first.

Local Exercise Groups

They are another effective way to help you get into your regular habit. It's a well understood fact that people who train in a group are more likely to maintain their activity longer than those who train alone.

Individual Exercisers

These are anyone who is prepared to get their head down and work out on their own. I applaud you. If it suits your work pattern and you prefer your own company this is often the best position to be in. You have control of your time, budget and results, so go for it. All you need is a program, some kit and the determination to achieve. I can supply a workout or design a programme especially for you, contact me by email exerciseplan2000@gmail.com

Plan To Work Out At Home

The following equipment may be of help to you; - keep it simple, but make it effective:

A set of suspension straps. There are a number of good suppliers to choose from in the UK www.monkeybargym.co.uk and the USA www.trx.com
A skipping rope
A 3kg medicine ball
A sandbag
Kettlebells; sizes vary enormously and depend on your experience.

They start at 4kg in weight and go up above 32kg. Go to a good supplier as there are a lot of poor quality copies on the market.

I would advise anyone to purchase from a reputable equipment supplier and beware when purchasing off the internet and cheap high street shops. If it's cheap avoid it. I would recommend www.dragondoor.com but there are many to choose from.

Choosing a Kettlebell

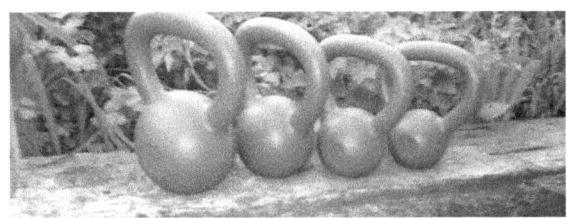

Choosing the right kettlebell can be confusing. My advice would be to keep to mainstream suppliers and avoid all the cheap imitations or copies you can find on popular online stores. These will ruin your training experience and they are generally poorly made; some with weird designs and can be plastic with handles which you may find will not allow your hand to glide through the movement easily.

The best kettlebells are cast iron with plenty of room in the handle for your wrist. Avoid buying anything too light as you will quickly find that as your technique and strength improves they may become too light and end up propping open the door.

Kettlebell Weights to Choose:

Between 8kg (18lb) and 16kg (35lb) for women,
Between 12kg (26lb) to 20kg (44lb) for men.

You will probably start with a lighter weight for upper body exercises such as the shoulder press, snatch and clean. Use the heavier weights for your swings, squats etc. I find that most clients quickly build confidence and find that using a heavier bell will improve their technique in all the moves.

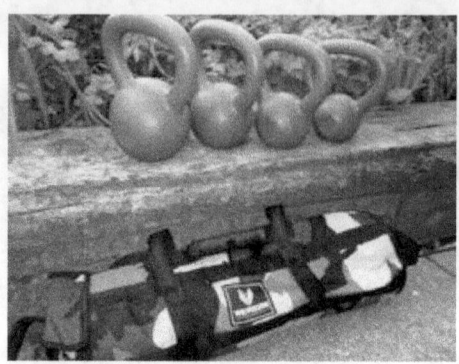

You can purchase the larger diameter competition bells made of steel. These have a larger bulkier design making them much more comfortable in use, stable for exercises such as push-ups and renegade rows, and less likely to bang up your arms while you are working on your technique.

To summarise; I advise at least two bells of different weights as you improve add another heavier kettlebell to your collection. Always choose quality over price even if you have to save for a while.

Personal Training

Engaging the services of a personal trainer is a good idea, especially if you wish for success, motivation, structure, and an education for life. It's most efficient for people who are not into or can't get to a Crossfit or Boot Camp group.

The first stage, when you are looking for a personal trainer, is to make sure they are registered and qualified through the "Register of Exercise Professionals."

In the UK you can use www.exerciseregister.org

In the USA there is a number of certification bodies
https://www.nasm.org   www.acsm.org/certification

Search in your country and you should get to a section for a search in your area. Read through the list and qualifications to search for trainers in your area, then you can check out (investigate!) their Facebook and websites for all the information you need to help you compile a short list of possible trainers.

I would also recommend that you ask friends for their advice and recommendations before booking a trial session.

Personal trainers are all different and finding one which suits you may take a little work, but will be well worth it. You are entering into a relationship with your trainer and may become firm friends as a result. As the saying goes; "choose your friends carefully."

"I think if you exercise, your state of mind - my state of mind - is usually more at ease, ready for more mental challenges. Once I get the physical stuff out of the way it always seems like I have more calmness and better self-esteem."

Stone Gossard

Suitable Clothing

They should be comfortable for the training environment and do not need to be the latest designer clothing. You can get started with a top, shorts or tights and trainers. See how you get on as you will soon work out what works best for you. In my experience you will want to buy something different, very quickly, from whatever you start with.

My closet is full of training clothes collected over the years. It's all good and I hate to throw things away (being financially and environmentally conscious), but I always want to buy a new set for each season. I have more trainers, jackets and backpacks than I know what to do with.

For tops, you do not need to be technical as you are probably only going to wear it for an hour and it will feel great when its soaking with sweat, as you will know if you have worked hard enough.

If it's dry at the end of your session, have you put in sufficient energy and determination? You have to put the effort in to sweat. Sweating means you are burning off calories.

Warming Up

This is something nearly everyone neglects. Whatever you do, do NOT neglect warming up, whatever age you are, and this becomes even more important as you enter one of the older age brackets. It is also the one area that when avoided, increases your risk of injury.

Unfortunately, most people just don't understand why you warm up or how to do it, they get in from work change and jump straight into their routine with only a rudimentary consideration of their warm up, by kicking their legs around followed by a couple of stretches - and they're done.

They may even jump on a treadmill, ergo trainer, upright gym bike or rower in the gym for 5 minutes and consider their warming up is complete.

People, please this is so wrong! This is your remedy for injuries like muscle fatigue turning into strains and even more serious, ruptures or complete fractures.

The Benefits of a Warm-Up Routine

To prepare your brain, body and joints for the exercise you have planned in your workout or activity, this entails performing a range of movements to warm up the muscles, lubricate the joints, which allow you to move fluidly as your body moves oxygen around your body to your muscles. You will get better results with less risk of injuries, which if sustained, will stop you training for weeks or months, in some cases.

How to Warm Up Properly

This process is what we describe as movement preparation by preparing your mind and body, using a structured approach, utilizing effective exercises in mobility from low level, to gradually warm up of the muscles and joints.

As you gently move the joints you lubricate them with the body's own synovial fluid, which is secreted as the joints are mobilized.

As you do this you are also gently pulling or contracting and stretching the various muscles attached to each joint, increasing blood flow; consequently warming them up.

Once warmed up they become more pliable and less prone to damage. (Stiff joints and cold muscles cannot easily cope with a lot of vigorous activity.)

Mobility

Mobility is our body's ability to move in all of the directions that we are supposed to - and need to move without restriction. Having proper mobility is important and necessary for good exercise techniques.

The ability for the body to move in all directions easily is the key here. If your body is stiff, your range of movement is limited. When you do something outside of that range your body will strain and you will suffer with a sore back, hip, groin or worse; perhaps a combination of all of those pains.

Stability

This is your ability to control your body against outside forces.

Your stability will be crucial, so practice each exercise with a range of light efforts within a comfortable range, to prepare the muscle groups for a gradual increase in work load, to prevent you from over loading the muscles.

Typical areas of concern will be to look for are squatting down to your knee. If you are unable to do this you will overload your back (for example, when lifting a heavy weight from the floor, e.g. washing machine, sofa or anything you don't usually lift.)

Where your knees cave in when squatting, this indicates a weakness around your knees, hips, abductors or glutes and requires gradual strengthening over a period of time. How to do this is something to ask your personal trainer or expert about, as it will be specific to your personal needs.

Choice of Warm Up

Each sports activity has its own unique set of mobility exercises. Follow these for 15-30 minutes before a game to be properly warmed up. At the end of a game, do some more light mobility to warm down and reduce the amount of muscle waste in the muscles, which increases blood lactate. This will make you stiff, if not removed.

General Mobility Examples

Where you are unsure what any of these mean, ask for expert guidance before you try to carry out these activities, to ensure you're completing them correctly.

Let's start at the top and work down to cover a total body warm up.

Head: Perform around 8 repetitions of the following:
Turn from side to side fully look over your shoulder
Push your chin forward, and back.
Then do circles with your head imagine you are drawing a circle with a pencil in your mouth.

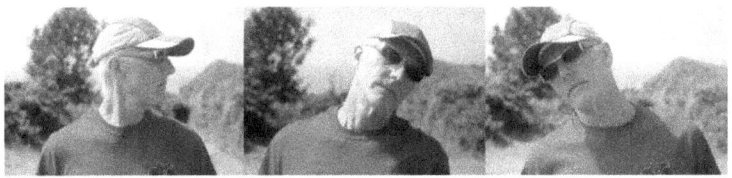

Hip bends maintain a flat back and bend forward hinging from the hip

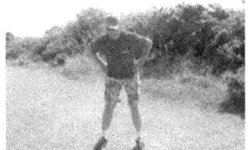

Side Bends push your hands down one side of your outer leg as far as you can, then repeat for each side.

Torso twists hold your arms parallel to the floor and sweep around allowing the opposite hip to follow lightly, perform on each side

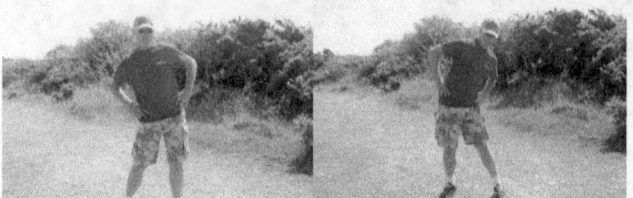

Toe touch one leg forward at a time L/R bending from the hips to reach the front of your trainers

Toe touch to the outside of the foot L/R

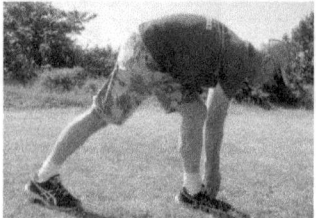

Leg swings to forward and back/ sideways/ across the Body/ over & unders

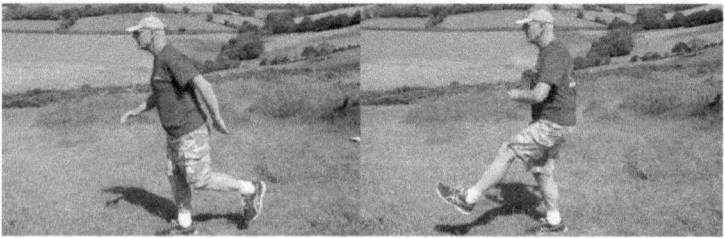

Squats with a floor touch L/R

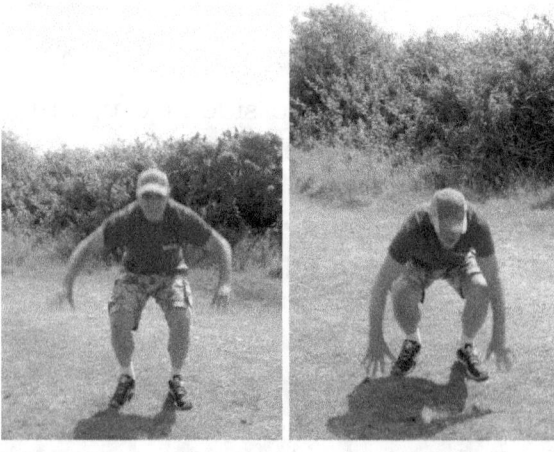

Push up / Burpee

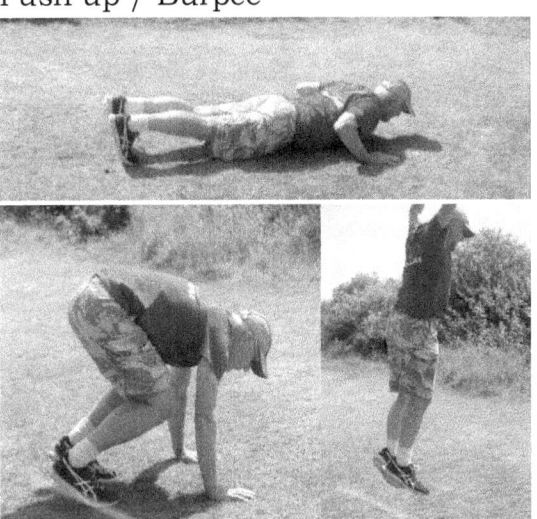

Hindu press ups

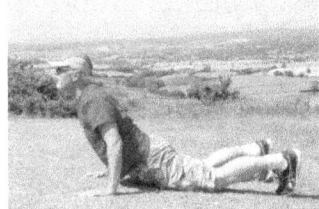 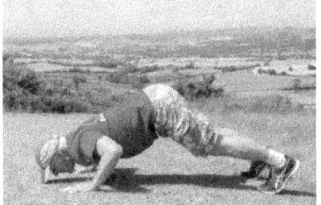

Hip raise to bridge

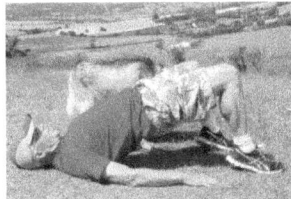

Multi direction Lunges

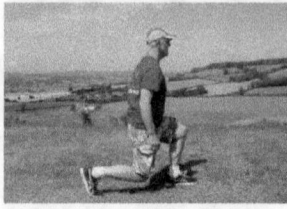

Skipping or jogging on the spot

Short sprints with floor touch

Performing most of these for around 20 seconds each, through 2 or 3 times, preferably with a partner to make it more fun. This will properly prepare your mind and body for your work out.

Ideally these exercises should flow through from one to the other so you are moving fluidly, gradually building up to a breathless state.

See Me in Action on My YouTube Channel

Please go visit my YouTube website pages where I provide some demonstrations of exercise and techniques which may help you. If there are any you want me to add, please just ask and I'll film the most popular requests:

Search for: **Exercise demonstrations by Norman Brown**

How to Stay Fit When You're Away From Home

This one is one of my favourites because I am always being asked this question. It is much simpler than you think, even if the hotel you are in does not have a gym.

First, you are either on holiday (relaxed) or on business (tough).

You will need a short 10 – 30 minute workout to generate that feel good factor to reduce the guilt you feel from being away from your usual routine.

Tools available to think about taking with you:

1. Skipping jump rope
2. Trainers and running kit
3. Swim costume
4. Suspension trainer to hang from the hotel door or a nearby substantial anchor point, around 6' to 9' high.
5. An empty sandbag you can fill with sand from the beach! I do this.

None of this will weigh much to worry about and it's all instantly available.

The reason for choosing these is based on your need for convenience, but they are also powerful conditioning tools when used in the right safe manner.

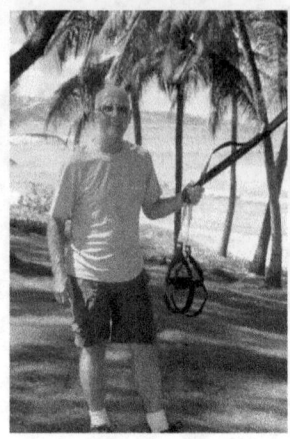

(I should use this photo of me with my suspension trainer, fit for trees as well, for the book cover. Oh, I did!)

Skipping is an excellent way to improve your cardio vascular fitness. It is light and weighs very little.

A sandbag is my tool of choice for conditioning and strength training. It is completely flexible, allowing you to add or remove weight, dependent on the routine you choose.

Most Common Exercising Mistakes

Here's a list of the most usual and often experienced difficulties:

1. Attempting to much too soon

2. Not having a health check

3. Not taking professional advice

4. Copying complicated techniques from You Tube

5. Copying what others are doing in the weights room

6. Using poor technique, particularly when weight training

7. Not recording your progress

8. Expecting amazing results and eating a poor diet – expected results won't happen.

9. Not putting the effort in

10. Refuelling with rubbish (fast food/sugar drinks soda pops) after your workout

Did You Know?

1lb fat = 3500 calories

The average cardio vascular workout = 500 calories per hour

"The reality is you have to improve your diet to make a real difference. Exercise helps, but is only part of your solution to losing weight."

"Our growing softness, our increasing lack of physical fitness, is a menace to our security."

John F. Kennedy

Exercise Routines

I'm a personal trainer and I can write a plan for you to follow. However, without knowing all about you I would only be guessing the routine and it would not be specific to your needs, muscular imbalances or health issues. In your own interest AND to avoid any potential litigation I am not going to encourage you towards any particular training plan, without knowing much more about you first.

The following thoughts are only ideas. They are examples of what you can do in certain situations with particular equipment and tools and in these cases I have illustrated routines which I use with my own clients including a number of other sources. If you want to talk through my personal choices for you specifically, we should arrange to meet, professionally, either by email or skype me.
exerciseplan2000@gmail.com

Fitness or Weight Loss Routine

I want to keep this as simple as possible and at the same time, making it an effective routine you can vary with practice.

You will use what we describe as compound exercises, which means using more than one muscle group in the same exercise; this is more effective due to the greater number of muscle fibres activated during the movement.

This provides a stimulated effect on your metabolism which will probably take all day to fully recover; burning off more body fat during recovery.

You can of course make this a more challenging work out by simply increasing the weights you are using and reducing the repetition range to around 5-8.

Use 15 repetitions and complete 3 – 5 sets depending on your fitness.

Choose one exercise option from those listed below:

Squat / Shallow / Deep past knee's
Overhead press / 20lb bar / Olympic bar / Kettle bell / Sandbag
Lunge / Forward / Side / Reverse
Using a hand weight like a sandbag or ball, lunge and twist towards the front leg
Chest press / Push up
Dead Lift / Straight leg / Single leg
Combine the dead lift with a push up and you have a similar exercise to a burpee without the jump.
Row / Seated / High / Fat boy / assisted pull ups
Torso twists / Russian twists / Cable twists / Bag around the worlds
Stability – Full Plank held for 15 – 60 seconds. Work on it!

Vacation or Business Routine

The most effective way to approach these workouts is by using High Intense Interval Training (HIIT). You can do this in 10 minutes to 30minutes. The best time is in the morning early before it becomes too hot and before breakfast; setting you up for your day.

Each routine should include a few minutes of mobility preparation.

Swimming

Workout 1

5 x 50m sprint freestyle (change strokes as desired)
Rest for 20 seconds (hydrate if needed)
5 x 100m sprints -- any stroke
Rest 40-60 seconds
The remaining time of your hour, swim at regular pace
non-stop for 15-30 minutes

Workout 2

Repeat 5 times
Swim 100-200m moderate pace
Push-ups - 30 seconds worth of push ups (10-40 reps
depending on fitness level)
Abs of choice - crunches, flutter-kicks, leg raises - 1:00 of
abdominal exercises
Workout 3
Repeat 5 times
Swim 100-200m moderate pace
Push-ups - 10-20
Crunches - 20-30
Bicep Curls - 10-20 reps
Shoulder Press - 10 reps

Jog/Running

Workout 1

Pick out a route of around 5k and do the first loop nice and easy.
On the second loop put in 200 meter increasing speed efforts with enough recovery to take on liquid
Push the last 500 meters back to hotel.

Workout 2

Warm up - 10 to 15 minutes of light jogging
Run 800m at race pace
20 Burpees, 20 push-ups, 15 single leg squats, both legs
30 crunches
Run 800m at race pace
20 Steps ups to high step L/R
20 Tricep dips
20 Lunges L/R
15-20 double crunches
Run 800m at race pace
20 squat to presses, 20-30 supermans
Run 800m at race pace
Cool down - 15 minutes of easy jogging, long stretching emphasis on Quads and hamstrings

Workout 3

1. Tempo intervals six minutes brisk, one-minute walk, six minutes brisk, one-minute walk, six minutes brisk.
2. Hills are also an excellent way to start your speed work. Try 6 x 1 minute uphill, jog back down. Gradually add extra reps until you can complete 10.
3. Add some fartlek (speed play) training to your schedule

To begin, try just a 25-minute run with quick bursts mix up the speed pace between slow/medium/fast

All Over Fitness and Conditioning

In this work out I have included a routine from the manufacturers of the suspension training system. Suspension training straps which promote the use of your body weight to develop strength in all muscle groups in a coordinated natural set of movements. I have added a more detailed description for these exercise routines as these may not be so familiar to you.

Sandbag Training from the Ultimate Sandbag Training Company.

Perform the following as a circuit, rest 45-60 seconds between exercises and then proceed to the next exercise. Perform three to five rounds as needed.

Circuit A

Power Clean+Front Squat+Press x 5
Good mornings x 15
Overhead Lunge x 6
Shoulder Get-up x3 per side

Circuit B

Single Leg Deadlift x 8 per side
Clean and Press x 5
Shovelling x 20
Bent-over Row x 12
Bear Hug Walks x one minute

Circuit C

Shoulder to Shoulder Lunge x 6 per side
Half Knee Shoulder to Shoulder Press x 8 per side
Bear Hug Squats x 12
Around the Worlds x 15 per side

Combo Workout 1

20 meter sprint
10 Burpee's
Repeat 5 times
20 meter sprint
10 Bodyweight squats
Repeat 5 times
20 meter sprint
10 mountain climbers
Repeat 5 times

Combo workout 2

10 burpees
40 seconds Mountain climbers
10 burpees
40 seconds Push ups
10 Burpees
40 seconds Step ups (20 seconds L/R)
Take 15-20 seconds rest in between each exercise if you
need it. Repeat 2 – 3 times

Skipping

15 minutes broken into 60 seconds of work with 15 seconds recovery, increase the work time the fitter you are and vary the technique to keep it interesting.

Basic jump or easy jump
Alternate foot jump (speed step)
Criss-cross, Side Swing, Over and Unders

"My wife and I work out together almost every day. It's just a great way to spend time together. We're going to run a marathon together later this year, and that's one more goal that we'll accomplish as husband and wife."

Bill Rancic

Record Your Start Point and Your Progress

Use a Fitness Diary

(copy/print these as diary pages, keep in a folder for regular competition)

Stats	Today	Month 1	Month 2	Month 3	Month 4
Date started					
My Stats					
Weight					
Height					
Measurements					
Waist					
Hips					
Chest					
Thigh					
Calf					
Total					
Run 1 mile time					
Distance in 10 minutes					
Push ups in 1 minute					
Pull ups in 1 minute					
Burpees in 1 minute					

Record Your Fitness Activity

Use Your Daily Diary - Record - What Actually Happened

Day:
Date:
Time:
Activity:
Weather:
Feel:
Distance:
Duration:
Pace/effort:
Heart rate:

You can look back and compare the reason why your performance varied.

Did the weather affect your training?
Are you always achieving more on a Tuesday, or perhaps on Sunday?
Which activities are best for you?
Which activities do you need to work on to increase your overall performance?
Which do you enjoy the most and is this reflected in your performance?

Consider the effect of your lifestyle and on your training, adjusting your lifestyle activities to have a beneficial effect on the training outcome. For example, if you are partying tonight you might want to move your usual morning session to later in the day, allowing more time to recover.

If you find yourself scheduled to work late try and arrange a morning training session.

Going to a BBQ at the weekend? Get a hard training session in before, to help burn off those extra calories to boost the benefits of eating extra protein.

"15 minutes a day! Give me just this and I'll prove I can make you a new man."

Charles Atlas

List Your Major Achievements

Day:	
Date:	
Time:	
Activity:	
Feel:	
Distance:	
Duration:	
Pace/effort:	
Heart rate	

For example:

I ran for 10 minutes without stopping

Completed my first 10min mile

My waist size dropped 5cms / 2"

My resting heart rate is lower in the morning than it was when I started training. For example, it used to be 85 it's now 70 or lower.

Clothing size changes

Training 4 times a week regularly instead of 2

Completed 3 mile, or 6 mile run in a certain time.

Beginner Training

Start with:

A walk or jog 20 – 30 minutes a day
Attend a group class 1-2 times a week
Record your activity and how you feel.

Two simple rules apply:

1. **Progress** your time excising by **10%** a week.

2. **Incorporate** exercise in to your daily lifestyle, so it becomes **part** of your routine.

Energy Expenditure

The amount of energy used during exercise varies according to the individual. In general, around 80 calories are burned every 10 minutes. This varies according to a number of factors such as your weight, fitness, the intensity of exercise and your choice of activity, determining the number of muscles used.

The less stress your body is under, the fewer calories you would use, due to the more buoyancy or support being provided by the activity, such as cycling, swimming or using the cross trainer.

It's important to remember that the energy used during exercise is from your stored glycogen kept in the muscles and the liver. Glycogen is produced by the liver, converting carbohydrates eaten and stored in the muscles and will last you for around 2 hours. Any surplus glycogen will then be stored inside the body as fat.

I am not an advocate of concentrating on counting calories out as these can be misleading and results are too short sighted. You are better to put in the effort you can and look to other more reliable means to measure your success, such as the measurements we mentioned earlier and - can you get into those trousers or the dress you were longing to get back into?

"Looking good and feeling good go hand in hand. If you have a healthy lifestyle, your diet and nutrition are set, and you're working out, you're going to feel good."

Jason Statham

For those who want to see how many calories you may target to burn, the following table will help.

Activity (1-hour duration)	Weight of person and calories burned (Choose whichever closely matches you)		
	160 pounds (73 kilograms)	200 pounds (91 kilograms)	240 pounds (109 kilograms)
Aerobics, high impact	533	664	796
Aerobics, low impact	365	455	545
Aerobics, water	402	501	600
Backpacking	511	637	763
Basketball	584	728	872

Bicycling, < 10 mph, leisure	292	364	436
Bowling	219	273	327
Canoeing	256	319	382
Dancing, ballroom	219	273	327
Football, touch or flag	584	728	872
Golfing, carrying clubs	314	391	469
Hiking	438	546	654
Ice skating	511	637	763
Racquetball	511	637	763

Resistance (weight) training	365	455	545
Rollerblading	548	683	818
Rope jumping	861	1,074	1,286
Rowing, stationary	438	546	654
Running, 5 mph	606	755	905
Running, 8 mph	861	1,074	1,286
Skiing, cross-country	496	619	741
Skiing, downhill	314	391	469
Skiing, water	438	546	654

Softball or baseball	365	455	545
Stair treadmill	657	819	981
Swimming, laps	423	528	632
Tae kwon do	752	937	1,123
Tai chi	219	273	327
Tennis, singles	584	728	872
Volleyball	292	364	436
Walking, 2 mph	204	255	305
Walking,3.5mph	314	391	469

(Adapted from: Ainsworth BE, et al. 2011 compendium of physical activities: A second update of codes and MET values. Medicine & Science in Sports & Exercise. 2011;43:1575.)

Once your workout has finished your body will recover by using up your fat reserves, by converting the fat back into glycogen and putting it back into the muscles.

This process will be completely wrecked if you go and have a post workout recovery cappuccino or any food containing carbohydrate, too soon after exercise. If your goal is to lose fat you should *definitely* take this <u>important note</u> into consideration.

"If your exercise is less than an hour, you do NOT need to drink sugary sports drinks. Water will be all you need."

If your aim is to improve fitness and losing high body fat is not the main goal, then you should refuel with a protein carbohydrate balance appropriate to your activity. Always consider that your body requires energy in balance.

As your activity levels increase over several hours in one session you will need to increase your carbohydrates to sustain this. If your interest is to increase muscle weight you will need to increase your protein intake and keep your carbohydrate intake moderate.

Nutrition Introduction

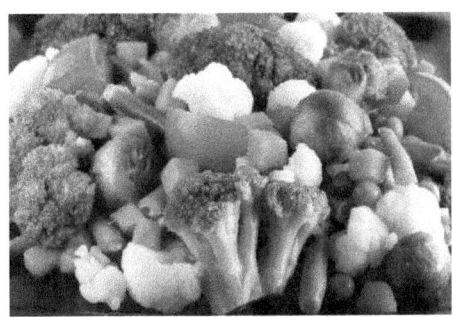

Food is the basis of your very existence and to abuse it is to abuse your body. In an age where convenience seems to be ruling every decision we take, you cannot be forgiven for ruining your body by making poor food choices.

We all like a treat and there is nothing wrong in that until... the treat becomes a daily habit. Your body will begin to suffer the strains of a modern diet laced with sugar, trans-fats and additives.

Your gradual increase in weight will be demonstrated as your waist line stretches; lethargy overtakes you, you have an obvious loss of energy, poor skin conditions, slow healing and high stress levels. Your cholesterol and blood sugar both becoming raised - then your blood pressure rises! Consequently, there is an elevated risk of all known diseases and higher levels of cardiac (heart related) incidents.

General Guidance

If you want to get the best out of your body you have to eat as well as you can within the budget available.

"You are what you eat"

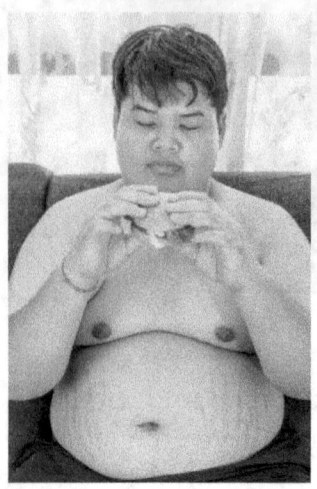

Your diet will determine your levels of energy, sleep, how quickly you recover after illness, the risk of developing cancers and cardio vascular disease, etc.

If you already have complications like this you may want to consult a nutritional therapist who is best qualified to advise you on specific conditions because my advice is going to be more generalised.

Why Nutrition Is Important

Your diet should be as fresh as possible with limited processed foods involved. Processed products have a higher level of additives with low nutritional content, leading to all the problems we are seeing in an increasingly obese population.

If you deprive yourself of sufficient nutrients your body will be unable to regulate your hormonal system which controls every aspect of your body's functions. You will see many references to individual conditions on the internet with advice on what to eat or not to eat. Importantly, they all share the same principle - your hormone system is out of balance.

Sleep, energy and repair processes are all controlled by your hormones.

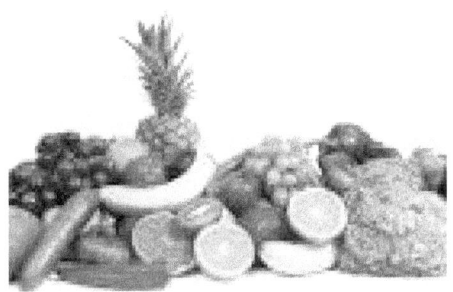

Your diet should high in vegetable and fruit sources of carbohydrate with moderate starchy carbohydrates such as potatoes, pasta, rice, pulses and grains. They should all be taken in portions relative to your energy levels with rich protein sources like meat, fish and dairy, eaten with your meals, at least three times a day.
Sweet items like dessert and confectionery should be consumed in moderation.

A little red wine and dark chocolate are good when taken in moderation as they are high in antioxidants which are required for cell repair.

Consuming plenty of fluids a day will help to improve your skin appearance and all of your body functions which require plenty of fluid. This includes tea, coffee, soups and anything which is nice and wet. Sensible recommendations are 8-10 glasses of water per day with an additional pint of water for each hour of exercise.

The Modern Food Pyramid - This is your target!

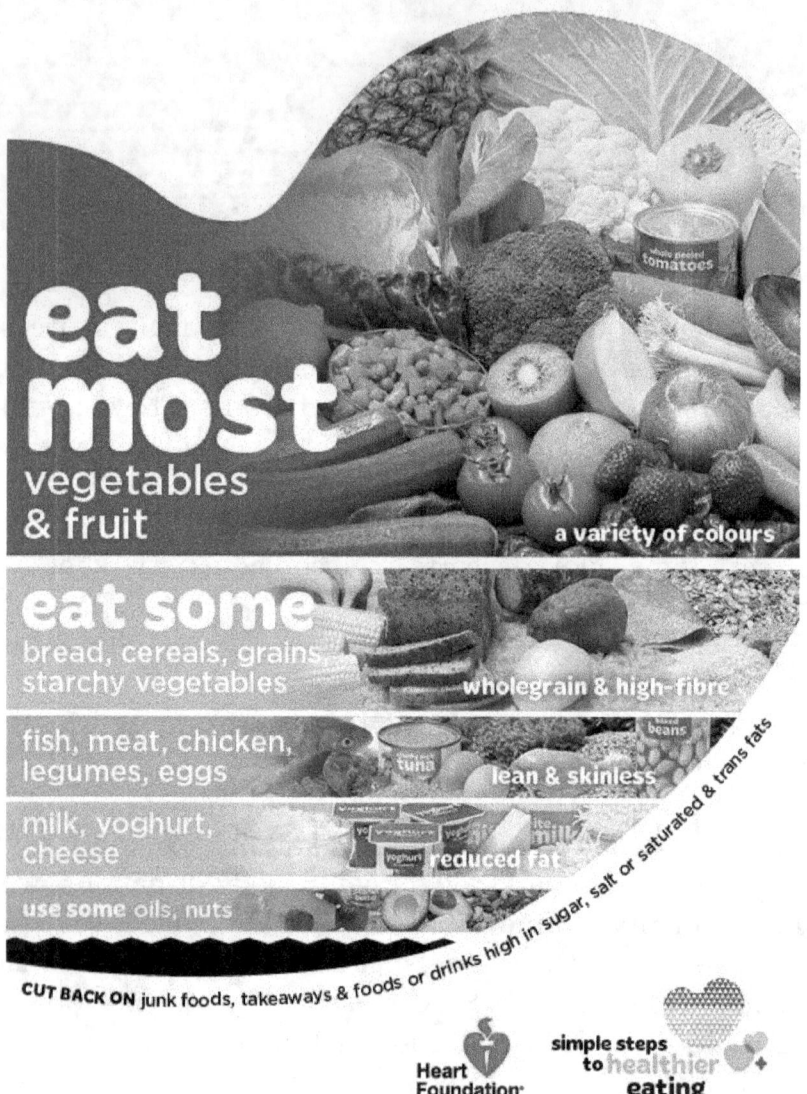

No Quick Fixes

There are no quick fixes if you are taken in by all of the advertising which claims pills and specific foods will help you lose body fat in a few weeks.

I urge you to resist wasting your money. Instead, invest in improving and eating a natural diet rich in colour and nutrients. If you have too, supplement with a good quality brand of suitable and appropriate multivitamins.

Why Diets Don't Work

Fundamentally, diets do not work over the long course and mostly you will end up in five years' time heavier than when you started your endless dieting.

Crash diets (where someone tries to quickly lose weight by cutting down on the amount of calories they eat) won't work for long-term weight loss and most aren't healthy.

Depending on the type of diet, it may slow down your metabolism (the rate at which your body turns food into energy). You can also prevent your body from receiving important nutrients and vitamins that your body needs to work properly, when you reduce your intake of carbohydrates (such as pasta, bread and rice), which are an essential source of energy.

It is better to increase your intake of protein and reduce processed carbohydrates at the same time consuming fresh fibrous fruit and vegetables.

It's Best to Lose Weight Gradually, In the Following Way:

1. At a rate of 0.5-1kg (1-2lbs) a week
2. By eating a healthy, balanced diet, combined with regular physical activity
3. By losing weight at a rate of 0.5-1kg (1-2lb) a week, you're more likely to maintain a healthy weight over the long term. Source [NHS]

Balancing Your Hormones

There are many factors affecting successful weight control. These lay in your ability to maintain a good hormone balance. Hormones are your chemical messengers which tell your brain what is happening within your body. When our hormones are functioning in harmony, they will measure your sleep cycles, controlling your body functions.

Where you regularly get less sleep than 7- 8 hours (for example; someone who works regular night shifts,) your hormone balance becomes disrupted, leading to an imbalance of leptin; higher cortisol, a stress hormone; ghrelin an appetite suppressant, insulin for sugar control, adrenalin, a stress hormone; resulting in tiredness, anxiety, irritability and food cravings.

Symptoms of low blood sugar can lead to an increase in body fat levels. Leptin will measure your fat levels and control when to store or release fat for energy and ghrelin controls your appetite - whether you should eat more. Sleeping less leads to an imbalance of these hormones with the result you will make unhealthy eating choices due to increased levels of ghrelin and store fat because of developing leptin resistance which causes higher levels of oestrogen which encourages the body to lay down more fat.

So you see, it's a vicious cycle. The only way to control these is to eat a well-balanced diet, low in simple sugars eating natural vegetables and fruit with a good source of protein.

Sleep maintaining 7-9 hours' sleep each night.

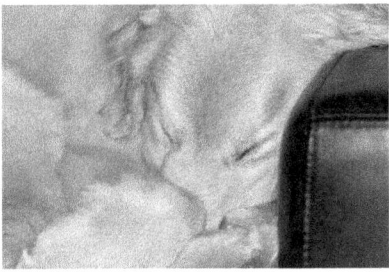

You are ready to sleep, generally when it starts to get dark, your sleep hormone, adenosine, will rise and your energy hormones, cortisol, will reduce allowing you to sleep normally. It is during your deep REM sleep that your body will regulate your hormones and help with body function repair. The long term disruption of good sleep will have a negative effect on this balance, causing a rise in a number of lifestyle risk factors. The principle impact is increasing the risk of developing type 2 diabetes.

Foods to Avoid and Why

Consuming any of the entire following list of foods, is basically increasing your risk of developing one or more of the most common lifestyle diseases. Source: [Mercola]

Canned Tomatoes

They are bad for you due to the high levels of Bisphenol-A, (BPA) - A Harmful Chemical used to line the cans and can be found in most plastic products, which can then contaminate the food which comes into contact with BPA.

This is a list of the potential health problems cause by prolonged exposure to BPA. Ref NIH

- reproductive harm
- increased risk of certain cancers
- malformation of organs in children
- risk of miscarriage
- sperm defects
- increased risk of mental disabilities in babies.
- hormonal disruption

Added Sugar and High Fructose Corn Syrup

You're probably not surprised to see sugar close to the top of this list.

In the last few decades, sugar has been considered as unhealthy because the calorific content is high, with no nutritional value.

That, however, is just the tip of the iceberg. New data links sugar to diseases that are killing people by the millions: obesity, diabetes, heart disease and cancers.

Artificial Sweeteners

There is an increasing opinion that sweeteners behave in the same way as sugar in that they have the same effect on the brain, by disrupting your metabolism and hormone balance, by increasing your tolerance to sugar, leading to increased abdominal fat storage, linked to obesity and type2 diabetes.

Sweetened Drinks

This includes diet versions. These are laced with artificial sweeteners or sugars and will increase your risk of obesity and some cancers.

These drinks can contain around 35 grams of sugar. Four grams equals one spoon of sugar. Do the maths; that's around 8+ tea spoons of sugar in each can.

Processed Meats

These include packaged hams, salami, sausage, deli meats etc. They are high in sodium (salt), saturated fats and preservatives. Consuming 50grams or 2oz a day can increase your risk of developing cardio vascular disease by 42% Source [Micha]

Convenience Condiments

These are found in abundance in all fast food and mall catering outlets. These are manufactured with preservatives to maintain a long shelf life. The preservative include food colouring, sweeteners, trans-fats and sodium. Eaten in abundance, they can increase your blood pressure and risk of CVD and cancer.

White Wheat Products

This includes shop purchased packaged bread, bagels, in-fact anything made with refined white flour. The refining process has removed all of the nutrients, vitamins and fibre from the wheat. Refined wheat products have been linked to inflammation, bloating and is also high in sugar.

Deep Fried Foods

Cooking food at high temperatures, particularly where it has been over fried, causes it to form toxic chemical compounds which when eaten, cannot be processed by the digestive system. Leading to an increase in LDL and decrease in HDL cholesterol, these increased levels of abdominal fat are linked with type 2 diabetes and coronary heart disease.

Seed and Corn oils

These fats have high levels of omega 6 fatty acids, where excessive consumption can lead to inflammation, cardio vascular disease and some cancers.

"Exercise to stimulate, not to annihilate. The world wasn't formed in a day, and neither were we. Set small goals and build upon them."

Lee Haney

There Are No Excuses for Failing to Eat Properly

Don't Use These Excuses – Ever!

Skipping breakfast

1. Too busy getting the kids ready for school
2. Getting up early for work and I don't have time
3. I have a slice of toast
4. Can't eat first thing in the morning
5. I don't need anything
6. I'll get a coffee and cake on the way to work

Skipping Lunch

1. Too busy at work
2. I eat at the desk
3. I have coffee and crisps
4. Grab a sandwich when I can
5. Nip out for a burger and a soda drink
6. I'm on the road so I grab a deli at the service station

You need to change these habits because they are making you fat and starving your body of energy during the day. This is a sure fire way to pile on weight because your body slumps into fasting mode and makes you tired during the day.

When you eat later at night your body stores this energy as fat.

Eating is supposed to be a social activity allowing you to socialise with family, friends and colleagues, during which your body can take time to digest and use the food you are enjoying for energy and muscle repair. This keeps your body in the shape it is designed for and evolved for.

My top tip for you if you have been making these excuses is to stop review and your schedule.

Make time to eat.

Enjoy meal time with family and friends. You will be amazed at how much better your life will feel when you do this.

"Physical fitness is not only one of the most important keys to a healthy body, it is the basis of dynamic and creative intellectual activity."

John F. Kennedy

Foods to Include In Your Meal Plan and Why

The best choice foods for every day health should be nutrient dense whole foods that you see in the market daily. They are easily available; bright in appearance and taste good.

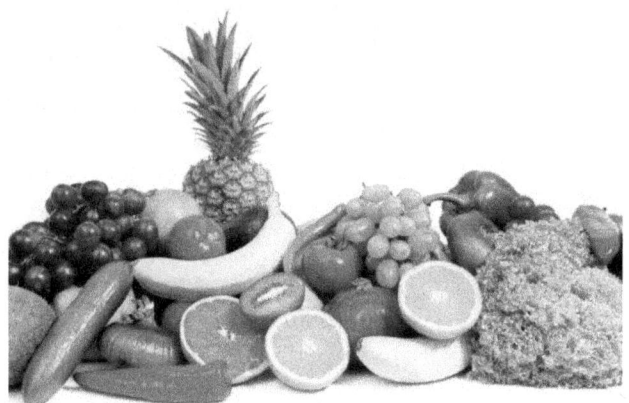

Ideally your food should have the minimum of processing, be natural, and where possible organic, for the maximum nutritional benefits.

How to Change From Processed To Fresh

Making eating habit changes is one of the most difficult things to work on. This is because there are so many associations between your lifestyle and your diet. If you recognised these associations we call them "triggers," because they trigger a behaviour that will call you to either grab something to eat or to sit in front of the television and crash.

Controlling your triggers is fundamental in achieving control over your energy levels, cravings and losing fat. When you feel the urge to crave, this is a clear sign your blood sugar is out of balance and falling, the last thing you should do is grab a quick fix candy bar or a shot of caffeine. This trigger needs controlling by improving your diet and eating sensibly.

You are unlikely to want to change to dramatically because this will probably elicit a shock to your body that you can't cope with and set you up for a fail before you start.

Make one or two changes you feel you can manage and keep these up until you are ready for another. Taking your time and creating change will be more successful over the long term. Two which are good to start with are eat breakfast and exercise 30 minutes every single day.

Watch for changes to your mood and energy levels as they improve. You should then be ready for the next one; let's say, eating more vegetables and reduce shop bought ready meals. You are going to notice that you naturally want to drink more fluids as you are exercising more.

Body measurements will start reducing as your fat reserves melt away and your cravings subside. This will feel great: you are now beginning to see that those lifestyle changes being accomplished though the successes you have now achieved.

Wanting to do this is something which has to come from deep inside you. Examine; do you want to; can you; why do you want to do this; what is pushing your button? You need to know this. Without understanding the reality of your needs, you will not succeed.

If you have the support of your family and friends, you are much more likely to overcome any obstacles. Their support may just be in sharing your experience with that acknowledgement that you are doing well and not policing you when you decide you deserve a treat. A simple well done, or you look great, is all that's needed sometimes.

Planning and Organization is important too. You need to organize these changes to make the process of change work.

What time will you train? What can get in the way and do you have a plan B? You might decide to train early in the morning by getting up an hour earlier, or join a friend for a lunch workout. Either way, has it been arranged and planned? When the answer is yes, you will do it and do it well.

Cycle of Change

Study this diagram illustrating the cycle of change. Study each of the five stages involved and consider your reaction to each and how you deal with each one.

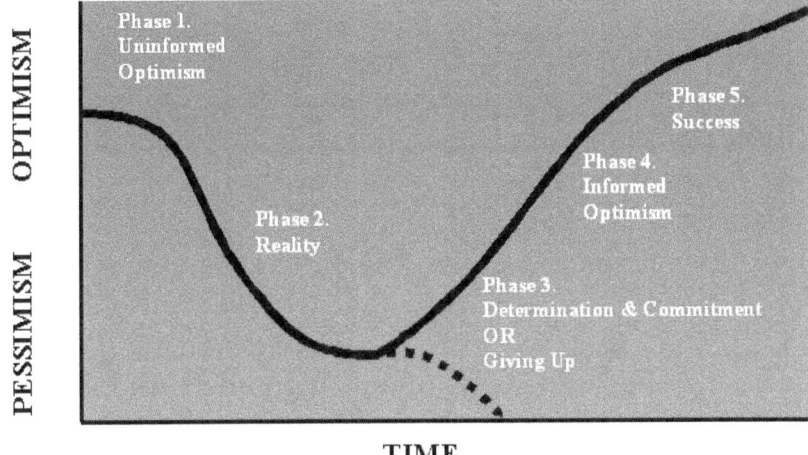

Organize Who Is Buying The Food?

Can you make some key switches to change from convenience to preparation of food, spend time with a friend or partner preparing your food for the work week, lunches, snacks etc.? This will help you always have a lunch and reduce any cravings for unhealthy choices from the coffee bar! This can be a very therapeutic experience in itself and research has proven that we are all much better people when we cook and eat together.

Eating is a social habit and when we eat with friends we are more likely to reduce stress and eat slower which will benefit the digestion process.

How to Make Fresh Convenient

If you don't cook, find a partner who does. This will make life much simpler. If you can't do that you will need to get adventurous and learn to cook.

Look for fresh ingredients like vegetables, salads and maybe fruits and start to mix them into salads or prepare them for snack boxes you can eat simply on the run, at work, or when travelling.

Bake your own flap jacks and make a smoothie with some protein powder you can easily take with you in a flask.

Buy a cook book and experiment with some simple quick bowl food or oriental recipes.

I suggest you avoid being too clever with complicated cook books - just keep it simple.

"Investing in early childhood nutrition is a surefire strategy. The returns are incredibly high."

Anne M. Mulcahy

How to Keep Going As You Get Older

What's older? If you are over 60 and been active for a number of years, like me, you will consider that age is only a number!

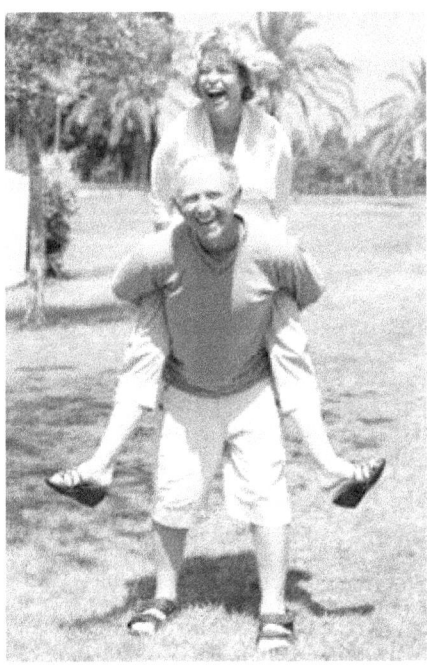

This might be true and there is plenty of evidence to suggest that your metabolic age may be 15-20 years younger than your actual age. As comforting as this is you can't and shouldn't deny the aging process.

The aging process in reality means you lose strength by as much as 70% compared to a young man. Your muscular structure will become less pliable and your bone density may decline. Ouch!

So, how to keep going tips:

1. Maintain daily activity

2. Vary your activity between some intensity and those of low intensity

3. Allow more time between hard activity sessions so you can recover. This will vary with the individual; between 2-4 days.

4. Take up Yoga or Pilates to maintain flexibility and good energy levels

5. Take massages frequently to maintain good muscle condition and tone, removing knots and tight adhesive muscle fibre

6. Drink plenty of fluid and reduce alcohol consumption

7. Sleep 9-10 hours for good recovery

8. Eat a fresh diet full of varied fruit and vegetables

9. Maintain good sources of protein from meat and fish unless you are a vegetarian. You need to find the best sources to suit you.

10. Take a good multivitamin - regularly!

A Summary of What You've Learnt So Far

You're On Your Way to a New You!

The point of this **Get Fit, Healthy and Staying That Way 40+** book is not to write a technical piece rather an introduction to remind you how easy it is and why you should exercise avoiding many of the pitfalls so many people trip up on; preventing them succeeding in their original goal to make a change.

You want to make a change right! So look through the passages which are relevant to you and prepare yourself to make whichever lifestyle choices which will improve how you feel about yourself. Take a photo every month to keep with your diary to remind you of your progress and where you have come from.

When you only have a couple of minutes spare to review parts of this book, please look over these summary thoughts first:

Stress, alcohol, activity, sleep, bone and muscle structure, exercise and diet.

Stress

Stress, particularly if it lasts long term, can have an adverse effect on your general health. Look for ways to reduce stress in your life if you are to avoid related health complications.

Alcohol

Drink alcohol in moderation. Excessive drinking can lead to several health concerns, so try to avoid a culture of over consumption. Excess may lead to weight gain or more serious social and health implications.

Activity

Stay active to reduce many health and wellbeing complications. Exercise has been shown to benefit:

1. Reduced stress
2. Maintain mental alertness
3. Reduced cardiac disease
4. Helps weight loss
5. Reduce risk of cancers.

Sleep

Improving sleep with 7-9 hours per night will provide an opportunity for hormone balance, providing a perfect environment for those chemical messengers to regulate all the bodies' functions.

It is important you look after your physical and emotional health in order to stay healthy and independent.

Otherwise, much of what you enjoy – perhaps gardening, playing golf or simply getting out and about – becomes that so much harder.

Maintain Your Structure

Bone is living tissue. As we age, the structure of bone changes and this results in loss of bone tissue.

Low bone mass means bones are weaker making them more prone to fractures.

Hormonal changes in women trigger the loss of minerals in bone tissue.

n men the gradual decline in sex hormones can lead to the later development of osteoporosis.

Muscles also lose significant levels of their strength as we age, which could lead to problems with moving about, and particularly with balance, leading to the potential of bone fractures.

Why Exercise?

1. Exercise can make bones stronger and help slow the rate of bone loss
2. Exercise increases muscle mass and strength
3. Exercise can improve balance and coordination and can help reduce the risk of falls
4. Exercise can give your mental health a boost; to combat anxiety, depression and stress
5. Exercise reduces your risk of cardio vascular disease and cancers and improves blood pressure
6. Exercise can improve blood cholesterol levels by increasing HDLs while lowering LDLs

Your Diet

1. Keep it simple.
2. Do not over consume if you are not exercising
3. Eat as fresh as you can manage
4. Eat lots of fresh fibrous vegetables
5. Eat fresh varieties of fruit and berries high in antioxidants
6. Eat moderate portions of meat or fish for protein
7. Eat smaller portions of refined carbohydrates for weight loss

I had an interesting conversation recently with a client who has lost 6 stone of body fat in the last few months. This conversation was an explanation of why the client was so fat in the first place.

It turns out that during adolescence they would often be sent to the shop to buy cheap food laden with sugar like ice cream for dinner, rarely having a good nutritious meal. This was not so much due to negligence, but poor parental education;

I would hope that this could not happen today, but sadly it does.

Today you should re-read this book before making a decision about how to approach any changes. Write down and plan what you need to do.

Complete your local research as to where to exercise, gain medical clearance and take all the measurements you need to evaluate your progress.

Keep a record of your diet over a few days, being honest. Don't cheat yourself; you are the only one affected. Where you see some obvious changes you can make to improve what you eat, make them gradually.

Often this may mean adding to your diet rather than taking away. In particular, water, vegetables, fruit, fibre and protein should all be included. Processed food, high sugar products, daily confectionary, alcohol and takeaways should all be minimised.

You are now ready to create a new YOU.

I want to wish you luck; I want to celebrate your accomplishments.

I want to give you support and guidance. You can email me personally if you'd like me to write you a programme, or provide online training exerciseplan2000@gmail.com

"NOTHING IS MORE SATISFYING THAN HEARING ABOUT YOUR SUCCESS."

References: Sources

Photo images courtesy of
http://www.freedigitalphotos.net/images/

Quotes courtesy of
http://www.brainyquote.com/quotes/topics/topic_fitness.html#YApMXCTvqgVlThiX.99

www.nhs.uk/Livewell/fitness/Pages/yoga.

http://www.plosone.org/article/info%3Adoi%2F10.1371%2Fjournal.pone.0109849

 http://chriskresser.com/the-diet-heart-myth-cholesterol-and-saturated-fat-are-not-the-enemy

http://www.diabetes.org/diabetes-basics/statistics/
2012 British heart foundation coronary heart disease statistics 2012
World Health organization
Energy expenditure chart by: Adapted from: Ainsworth BE, et al. 2011 compendium of physical activities: A second update of codes and MET values. Medicine & Science in Sports & Exercise. 2011;43:1575.
www.Mayoclinic.org
http://www.niehs.nih.gov/health/topics/agents/sya-bpa/
http://circ.ahajournals.org/content/121/21/2271
http://authoritynutrition.com/7-unhealthy-foods-to-avoid/
http://www.nhs.uk/chq/Pages/2468.aspx?CategoryID=51
http://articles.mercola.com/sites/articles/archive/2013/06/10/9-unhealthy-foods.aspx

You are what you eat image http://www.getskills.com/wp-content/uploads/2013/08/you-are-what-you-eat.jpg
www.Ultimatesandbagtraining.com
www.trxtrainingsystems.com

Please Look Out For My Other Fitness Books:

Back care exercises

Healthy heart

Glucose and exercise

Goal setting

Coping with stress

Flexibility

Team sports – pre-warm ups

"Take care of your body. It's the only place you have to live."

Jim Rohn

www.ingramcontent.com/pod-product-compliance
Lightning Source LLC
Chambersburg PA
CBHW072207280526
45788CB00002B/914